Dear S

we're all going on a summer holiday…
(blow the NHS!)

Len Bartholomew (LB)

A sequel to:

Dear Susan…don't drink and decorate…
(a blueprint for the NHS?)

Dear Susan is the secretary to three orthopaedic surgeons at St George's Hospital. Her contribution is recorded for posterity in the first 'Dear Susan…' paperback published on 13th July 2023 with heartfelt thanks.

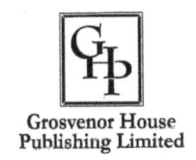

Grosvenor House
Publishing Limited

All rights reserved
Copyright © Len Bartholomew, 2024

The right of Len Bartholomew to be identified as the author of this work has been asserted in accordance with Section 78 of the Copyright, Designs and Patents Act 1988

The book cover is copyright to Len Bartholomew

This book is published by
Grosvenor House Publishing Ltd
Link House
140 The Broadway, Tolworth, Surrey, KT6 7HT.
www.grosvenorhousepublishing.co.uk

This book is sold subject to the conditions that it shall not, by way of trade or otherwise, be lent, resold, hired out or otherwise circulated without the author's or publisher's prior consent in any form of binding or cover other than that in which it is published and without a similar condition including this condition being imposed on the subsequent purchaser.

A CIP record for this book
is available from the British Library

ISBN 978-1-80381-872-6

Front and back covers – the beach and harbour wall, Greece – seen through rose tinted glasses (as is the NHS in this sequel!).

"Don't judge a book by its cover" – George Eliot

For Rosie (Rosemary (RG))

And for all those listed in the 'Acknowledgements and Epitaph (revised).' Many thanks to those involved in Nucleus (and its forerunners) for their talent and hard work. Also, thanks to the target audience for unintentionally providing the impulse for this sequel.

Foreword

I was surprised when I realised LB was writing a sequel to his previous paperback – published as recently as the 13th July 2023.

I thought that having extracted a large bee from his bonnet with his first paperback LB had done his bit and we could now get on with the rest of our lives! Especially as he had ended with "A Last Word."

I appreciate that LB's target audience had been a huge disappointment to him. Most of this audience has been unable to join him in a healthy debate about improving hospital buildings within which patients are treated and NHS staff have to work. So, perhaps it is hardly surprising that LB was intent on writing a sequel to reinforce his message.

I have to say that his b...... persistence is borne out of the unique position he held for a number of years in the 1990's, well aided and abetted by a large talented team of enthusiasts. Their task was to review the results of the hospital building programme from 1970 – 1990 and to look forward to make predictions about future provision. Also, since then LB has had to endure inpatient care in a large teaching hospital and put up with "the process imperfections." All this while the NHS estate has fallen into disrepair alongside a decline in services and a real dissatisfaction about the NHS's performance in caring for the health of the nation.

Covid inevitably worsened the slowdown in services and lengthened the queue to a free and accessible NHS. Could someone please do something to relieve those unfortunate patients on that interminable waiting list by sorting out the healthcare estate and let LB and me off the hook?

RG

February 2024

Preface

My first 'Dear Susan...' paperback described a possible blueprint for the NHS. This was set against a personal commentary about my recent experience as an inpatient in a large teaching hospital which highlighted some of the difficulties facing patients. It was intended as an easy read for a busy target audience sent complimentary copies in the weeks following publication.

It now seems it was not an easy read and that most of those targeted were too busy packing for their summer holidays to dip into this paperback before taking their leave. If staff in those offices of those targeted thought to hand a lightweight little booklet to their bosses as they left for their holidays it was likely to be left on some faraway shore. Maybe they were hoping the NHS will have sorted itself out on their return - as if by magic!

Perhaps the moral of this story is that one should avoid publishing a paperback like mine just as the summer holidays begin and on 13th July if superstitious.

Its cover photograph of a beach and harbour wall in Greece may have put off some readers not expecting a paperback looking like holiday reading to labour over a blueprint for the NHS. This was chosen to provide an image for Chapter 10 'The Great Escape - May 2022.' It had given inspiration to a non-ambulant patient who seemed at times to be going nowhere.

This sequel uses the same front cover with a modified title (for a tease). It now encloses a kind of review (a complaint really) about what happened following publication – or more to the point what did not happen. It shows how the target audience, including some people in a position of power, were simply too able to ignore a possible blueprint when there is a scarcity of blueprints.

It also provides me with a second chance to make a case for new smaller hospitals. This time using a few illustrations, even though the first 'Dear Susan...' had tactically not included any! All of this is in hope that there is someone out there savvy enough to want to try to build a brighter future and renew confidence in a hard done by NHS.

LB

February 2024

Contents

Introduction	1
Chapter 1 – The Target Audience	5
Chapter 2 – Once Upon a Time Around 1970 – The Millenium	13
Chapter 3 – We will build 40 New Hospitals – but not this week	27
Chapter 4 – Dear Select Committee	31
Chapter 5 – Dear Secretary of State	37
Chapter 6 – Enough is really Enough	41
Chapter 7 – Non – Fantasy Smaller Hospitals	47
Chapter 8 – A Healthier Population	53
Chapter 9 – Why so B..... Persistent	59
Chapter 10 – Epilogue according to LB	67
Acknowledgement and Epitaph (Revised)	69
Another Last Word	73

Introduction

LB has the impression that somehow it is too easy to dodge NHS issues that need to be tackled urgently because in no time the next crisis comes to the fore. Even with horrible headlines like those below, it no longer seems possible to provide the right kind of hospitals to help improve the health of the nation.

"Most people die while on NHS waiting list" - The Times - 23rd August 2023

Or to make the point again!

"The number of people dying while waiting for care is a national tragedy" Louise Ansari, CEO Healthwatch England – August 2023

Are the above headlines a good enough reason for publishing a sequel to a too little read paperback published only recently on 13th July 2023? Yes, there might just be someone more favourably placed to make a difference – if that someone can be nudged into reading and understanding its message.

Before this message can be developed further, perhaps there is a need to explain why the previous 'Dear Susan…' paperback was published in the first place.

INTRODUCTION

Maybe this is best answered by referring to the editor's report from its back cover. This in a nut shell, is one of the few encouraging reviews received. Encouraging because it is on message:

> ".... This was a really interesting insight into your experience and subsequent efforts to engage with a struggling NHS and suggest changes to improve the experience for future patients. I imagine the lack of adequate responses from various places must have been incredibly frustrating! Your passion is admirable and I share your hopes that something changes and our NHS can be functional again.......................
> ....I'm glad you are on the mend and hope you have lots more holidays lined up!" Polly Warren

Now you have this review in mind you have less need to buy a copy of the first 'Dear Susan…' paperback. It can be left on the book seller's shelf to gather dust. This sequel lifts and uses key passages to rerun some of the arguments promoting a blueprint for smaller hospitals. The previous personal bits about experiencing the NHS as an inpatient during Covid are now less important – LB's wound has nearly healed if not the memory. It is enough for the reader to know that LB experienced the NHS from the inside in a state of "shock- horror"

Some of the reused passages are tinkered with to introduce illustrations[1] in an attempt to re-present the case for smaller hospitals.

---

[1] For the first 'Dear Susan…' paperback LB decided not to include any designs and sketches apart from the one included in Chapter 10 - to lighten the story and for old times' sake. This was because he had found over many years that most people tended to turn a blind

DEAR SUSAN... WE'RE ALL GOING ON A SUMMER HOLIDAY...

This 'Dear Susan...' sequel again shows how frustrating it can get when people appointed to make a difference are not able to find time to read a little booklet/paperback as they travel to and from their office or when they go on holiday. Of course, it could be that the message or the messenger is the problem. However, it seems more likely that having to provide healthcare for an increasingly accident prone, unhealthy and aging population in an understaffed NHS with too many horrible hospitals is all too taxing for most of the chosen target audience to tackle[2]. Also. It must be irritating to have to read what a jumped up/falling down off a ladder decorator/patient/retired architect has to say in a cheap looking paperback – albeit with a nice holiday photo on its cover.

In the previous 'Dear Susan...' paperback it was suggested that if you ever happen to need inpatient care and the NHS is still in dire straits, you should make sure you have a supportive family WhatsApp Group and your own Dear Susan. They deserve another mention in this sequel. Dear Susan features again with many thanks in Chapter 1.

---

eye at the sight of a plan or drawing. He chose to play a word game to avoid a need for illustrations. It could be that a few illustrations might have helped an interested reader to stay the course and show in more detail how "Fantasy Smaller Hospitals" might be realised. LB has two fraying strings to his bow so why not use both words and doodles to try to hit his moving targets?.

[2] LB has discovered he is not alone in being ignored – see The Times Magazine of 30/12/23 which describes how two anaesthetists cannot find a way to replicate their "high intensity theatre strategy" nationwide after successfully introducing it at Guy's and St Thomas' NHS Trust to reduce the waiting lists.

INTRODUCTION

The WhatsApp Group 'don't drink and decorate' dutifully ordered copies. Dear Jane asked "it needs to be read by the right person. Who is that?" LB could only answer lamely that he could not think of a single addition to the target audience listed in Chapter 1 who might significantly be able to change the NHS from what it has become. It therefore does not bode well for this 'Dear Susan...' sequel!

Perhaps this is too defeatist? This sequel might just be more successful in hitting the target this time around. It seems worth one more try! In for a penny in for a pound - especially as £100's millions have been spent since the 1990's in anticipating what future hospitals might look like with the on rush of AI.

In 2020 Covid came to call to confirm a seed change was desperately needed – what further proof do we require?.

Chapter 1

The Target Audience

The list for the target audience is not too long:

Dear Susan and Mr Consultant – with many thanks.

Chair of St George's, Epsom and St Helier University Hospitals Health Group

Dear Chief Transformation Officer – St George's Hospital

Local District and GP Nursing Services

Dear Clare – South West London NHS

Secretary of State for Health and Social Care

Shadow Secretary of State for Health and Social Care

Former Chair of the Health and Social Care Committee 2020 – 2022

Current Chair of the Health and Social Care Committee – see below

Minister of Health – 1975 - see below

Medical Director – NHS England

Mole Valley District Council

The wrong type of Times columnist

An overworked BBC Health Editor + 2 BBC journalists

RIBA Publications

Architects for Health

President of the Royal College of Surgeons-England

THE TARGET AUDIENCE

So, what did this target audience make of the first 'Dear Susan...' paperback?. Not a lot! Some had something to say, some (most) chose to ignore it and remain silent. No one really felt able to address a hospital building led initiative let alone a plea for smaller hospitals. There was seemingly little interest in a possible blueprint that might take on board the lessons from Covid - even though this might lead to prioritising emergency care and day care to help reduce the massive waiting list facing the NHS. It is difficult to report on silence when deafening but such is the dilemma facing the NHS, it seems worth detailing some of the reactions that were received – none of which move the debate further forward. Some were interesting if not supportive.

Firstly, and most importantly an email from "Dear Susan" dated 31st July 2023:

Dear "Leonard"

Just wanted to drop you a line to say that I thoroughly enjoyed reading your book which was full of humour/ patience/tolerance and alas a grave insight at the poor state of the NHS. I can only agree with your observations/proposals and sympathise with your hospital experiences especially being an inpatient. My goodness – imagine being offered jelly and custard! That was definitely a NO!

After everything you have been through from your body covered in Elephants Breath to the delight of the paramedics and the intolerable uncomfortable frame on your leg you certainly deserve your holidays in Greece and swims to the harbour wall. Your perseverance and acceptance and of course the healing hands of the consultants have pulled you through ....

Fondest regards

"Dear Susan"

Secondly, and encouragingly, an exchange of emails with the Chair of St George's, Epsom and St Helier NHS Healthcare Group from 28th August 2023:

Hi Len

I read your book while I was away.

I agree about the need to invest in new hospitals in a planned and comprehensive way but not your preference for small ones. On the whole bigger hospitals have better outcomes and if we were starting from scratch we wouldn't put all hospitals where they are now.

It's academic I am afraid as there is no way we will get the money needed to sort out the hospital estate even under a new government, given the state of the public finances.

But thank you for thinking about it and caring – that is much appreciated.

And I am very pleased that despite the process imperfections, the care you received from St George's was good and you are pretty well recovered from what was obviously a very nasty break.

With every good wish

Gillian

THE TARGET AUDIENCE

Email to Chair of St George's from LB of 30th August 2023

Thanks Gillian

I hope you enjoyed your holiday.

I appreciated getting your email of 28th August. I have noted your comments. You are one of a few from my target audience who has taken time to dip into my paperback and to respond – even though you are one of the busiest.

I liken your role to that of an Admiral of the Fleet steering a mega convoy/Health Group towards a hurricane in choppy seas. Your huge listing flag ship with its rusting hull, NHS St George's, has in its wake a convoy of large ships – the St Helier followed by Epsom which is towing a new old-style NHS Sutton currently without an engine. Other vessels make up the fleet but these are bobbing out of control and are likely to sink without trace. Given the state of the public finances, what is needed is one or two (or more) state-of-the-art/ark tugs to turn the convoy towards calmer seas or a safe port but unfortunately for the time being St George's is not for turning!

As I see it, your fleet could do with a new, unsinkable, float alone, fully equipped and self-sufficient Trauma Centre tug which might temporarily be lashed alongside St George's (re my Chapter 5) or better still be cast off to take the Trauma Team to a dry dock (say for example, a site next to the M25's Cobham Service Centre to be on hand for the M3, M4, M40, Heathrow etc). Also, the combined St George's and St Helier renal crew might be air lifted from the convoy onto another new, unsinkable, float alone, autonomous Renal Centre tug dry docked in Surrey (re my Chapter 7).

And so on, to plan for priority specialities like a new elective care centre (a third tug) to replace your existing day surgery units – retaining the one at Epsom. This might float alone away from St George's which is to be gradually decommissioned and suitably located as and when a need is proven and funds become available.

None of this is academic but requiring speed of thought and movement – which is not usually available to the NHS. The two ideal sites (discussed in my Chapter7) have already been snapped up by opportunistic and quick-witted house builders – one of whom is already on one of these sites.

Who gives a damn about apathy?.

Thank you again – I will bother you no more.

Best wishes

LB

Email to LB from Chair of St George's of 31st August

Dear Len

We share the same objectives and frustrations!

All the best - Gillian

Thirdly and a real relief, an email from Minister of Health – 1975 dated 19th August 2023

Dear LB

I am so sorry not to have acknowledged your letter and little booklet before now. I put it to one side to dip into while I was away this month. I agree very much with you that hospital design is very important. Thank you for sending it to me.

Yours sincerely

David..........

THE TARGET AUDIENCE

It was pleasing to receive an acknowledgement from another of the target audience. Was LB able to take this to mean that the Minister of Health – 1975 was happy with the account in the first 'Dear Susan... Chapter 3' of what he and others were trying to do 'Once Upon a Time Around 1975' and that maybe it was time to try this again now? Probably not but never mind – at least this email did not contradict the reportage of that significant event.

Strangely, our paths nearly crossed at Kalamata airport in October 2023 as two queues converged at the boarding desk in the departure lounge. Minister of Health – 1975, looking slightly older, more fragile but more suntanned than LB, was totally immersed in his iPad reading out loudly to anyone who cared to listen details of the staggering number of Russian troops killed in combat in Ukraine! 50 years on, after many political and literary accomplishments, Minister of Health - 1975 can be forgiven for not wanting to go round LB's buoy again!

So, what about some of the others?

Former Chair of the Health and Social Care Committee 2020 – 2022 has gone on to greater things so can be excused from not having time – or can he?[3].

Current Chair of the Health and Social Care Committee; "Steve will endeavour to take a look if and when time allows" – 18th August 2023!

---

[3] At least LB and RG's written evidence to the HSSC was attached to its inquiry report 'Clearing the backlog caused by the pandemic' – published in January 2022 – see also this sequels Chapter 4

Shadow Secretary of State for Health and Social Care - "Due to Parliamentary protocol, MP's are unable to act on behalf of individuals who live outside their constituency" – automatic response from his parliamentary and constituency offices following numerous prompts. Eventually, Sam from the Parliamentary Office emailed LB on 19th October 2023 to say "I am writing to confirm that we have received a copy of your book and that Wes is very grateful".

Interestingly, LB came across a Times Editorial of 24th January 2024 that thought to look to the shadow secretary of state to reform the NHS (if/when elected). It seems shadow secretary was impressed by a slogan he saw pinned to a wall when visiting a hospital in Singapore which read "Get rid of Stupid Stuff." Maybe the shadow secretary of state would be in with a shout if he read a few paperbacks! His constituency office told LB that he receives hundreds of books every week and can't be expected to read them all!. LB wondered how many of these were offering up a blueprint for the NHS!.

NHS England – Medical Director's Office - "He is looking forward to reading this" – 11th October 2023.

The wrong type of Times Columnist - "...though it sounds interesting, I fear I'm not able to give your book the time it deserves in my busy schedule" – 18th September 2023.

LB is disappointed to end this chapter by reporting a nil return from most of the others on The Target Audience list. So, it is up to you whether you choose to continue

THE TARGET AUDIENCE

reading this sequel knowing that you may be entering a silent world. To do so you will need stamina, perseverance, time and to be able to resist turning a blind eye at the sight of a plan in order to understand its message.

What you do with the message is anyone's guess!.

Chapter 2

Once Upon a Time Around 1970 – The Millenium

Around 1970, The Minister of State for Health at the Department of Health was seeking action that might drastically reduce the time it was taking to plan and build new hospitals and prevent the massive time and construction cost overruns that were a common occurrence. Also, he wanted to know more about a programme of standardised hospitals for a rapidly changing and uniform NHS to replace the Victorian and pre-war legacies.

At that time, there was little thought given to the consequences of achieving rapid build hospitals and about how they might be managed and staffed. It was enough to show that it could be done. No one thought it would be possible to build hospitals faster than it would be to train or recruit staff or whether it would ever be possible to afford to replace all those hospitals that were no longer fit for purpose in a shorter time frame.

So, a discussion between the health minister, the chief works officer and the chief architect kick-started the largest ever, nationally controlled, hospital-building programme. Probably the largest building project of any kind anywhere apart from the Great Wall of China.

To tackle the task, a third of a central London skyscraper was used to house a team of over 150 doctors, nurses, administrators, researchers, engineers, quantity surveyors and architects. They were to focus their minds on delivering the nucleus hospital briefing and design system. They were assisted by teams in 14 regional health authorities across the country who would be responsible for commissioning nucleus hospitals in each region. Many private practice architects and engineers would design and arrange tenders for hospitals tailored to meet local service planning priorities. It was a huge undertaking using a simple planning concept. Standard hospital departments were planned in a cruciform template – hospital Lego blocks – that could be assembled to form the nucleus/part of a whole hospital. For example, four operating theatres, support rooms and a recovery ward were planned to fit into one cruciform template. This same template could house two 28-bed wards, and so on.

For new hospitals, a first phase 'Nucleus' might use 12-16 cruciform templates with six to eight on each of two floors, providing up to 300 beds. A hospital providing 300 beds, the size of a district general hospital serving a local catchment area of 250,000 people, could be expanded to provide up to 600 beds. The cruciform template, in rows either side of a hospital street, allowed for natural lighting and ventilation[4] and was intended

---

[4] In 1990, a low-energy nucleus hospital was show to use 50% less energy than older hospitals, helped by natural lighting and ventilation, and its cruciform templates.

to be used for two- and at most three-story solutions. The templates could also be used as an addition to an existing hospital.

The architectural profession loved or hated nucleus. Some practices resented only being commissioned to construct and elevate hospitals using standard data. Others were pleased to be informed about specialised aspects of hospital planning and design and contributed hugely to the provision of hospitals fit for rapidly changing treatment procedures. Prior to nucleus, the notion that each hospital should be unique and reflect a new opportunity to reinvent what a hospital should be had resulted in some being costly and unworkable – some have been demolished perhaps prematurely. Some nucleus hospitals were disappointing but others were inspirational. They all consistently worked for the staff using them.

In 1991, a published review indicated that 28 new nucleus hospitals had been commissioned. This type of hospital continued to be built for another ten years after the chief architect retired in 1993.

Ironically, or befittingly, the chief works officer and chief architect, who joined forces with the health minister to give birth to nucleus, both lived in Reigate and were to see out their last days in East Surrey Hospital, Redhill – one of the first nucleus hospitals to be commissioned. It was a close call for the decorator/patient/retired architect when he was transferred from the same local hospital to St George's Major Trauma Centre.

ONCE UPON A TIME AROUND 1970

Eventually over 150 were built of all sizes using the cruciform template, which, over time, was revised internally to incorporate changing standards. Of course, nucleus had its downside. Some of the nucleus hospitals built were too large, in the wrong place, and are now in need of upgrading. However, many of them are still much better than most of the one-offs built before or at the same time.

The Covid pandemic, the resulting chaos, and the need to clear a massive backlog of patient operations has left the NHS wanting a new generation of rapidly built hospital buildings. Unfortunately, there does not seem to be anybody around with a political will to make this happen.

Nucleus hospitals will serve the NHS for a few more years yet but they were not designed to deal with the backlog caused by Covid. Something different is needed to fix the NHS but it is not by building one or two mega-hospitals or by attempting to transform large existing hospitals like St George's.

In providing rapidly built nucleus hospitals in the 1970s, '80s and '90s, it was argued that these should replace or improve Victorian and pre- and post-Second World War hospitals when it might have been more appropriate to set out a new service plan for the nation's health care needs. Some nucleus hospitals were built alongside existing hospitals where it was soon clear that they should have been located elsewhere. However, from the conveyor belt of new nucleus hospitals, a few were set aside to be built to stand alone on newly acquired sites.

When this happened, it was possible to reflect on a new beginning for the NHS.

New, easy, fast, smart, smaller hospitals could provide the next generation of hospitals. All that is needed is for someone in the NHS to want to build one to shine the light in the current darkness. How this might work is dealt with later in subsequent chapters. It stems from a notion that would leave existing NHS hospitals as they are for the time being and to only build new hospitals specialising in either trauma emergency care – for which there seems to be an ever-present need – or elective care to efficiently deal with the waiting list backlog, handling procedures that can be done in a day. These would be self-sufficient stand-alone hospitals built quickly to cause an impact. Existing hospitals would continue to be used for all other specialties – upgraded where obvious.

In 1975 the health minister was trying to get a grip on building new hospitals in 'the difficult economic circumstances of the next few years[5]'. He was wanting to encourage the development and use of nucleus hospitals with a standardised but flexible basic design of around 300 beds. 'Large district general hospitals built in one phase were no longer feasible.' More fundamentally, he thought that 'by building for the essential, not the desirable, number of beds, one can spread the limited capital resources and start more new hospital development'. Also, 'in the absence of growth and the presence of high Inflation, capital restriction will be greater than anyone would wish over the next few years.'

---

[5] Extracts from a 1975 keynote speech made by the Minister of Health.

This look back at once upon a time around 1970 strangely fits the context of today following the Covid pandemic. It could also be argued today that we should not be building hospitals as large as 300 beds. Large hospitals are from the past and things need to move on – the decorator/patient/retired architect found his time at St George's a painful flashback.

DEAR SUSAN... WE'RE ALL GOING ON A SUMMER HOLIDAY...

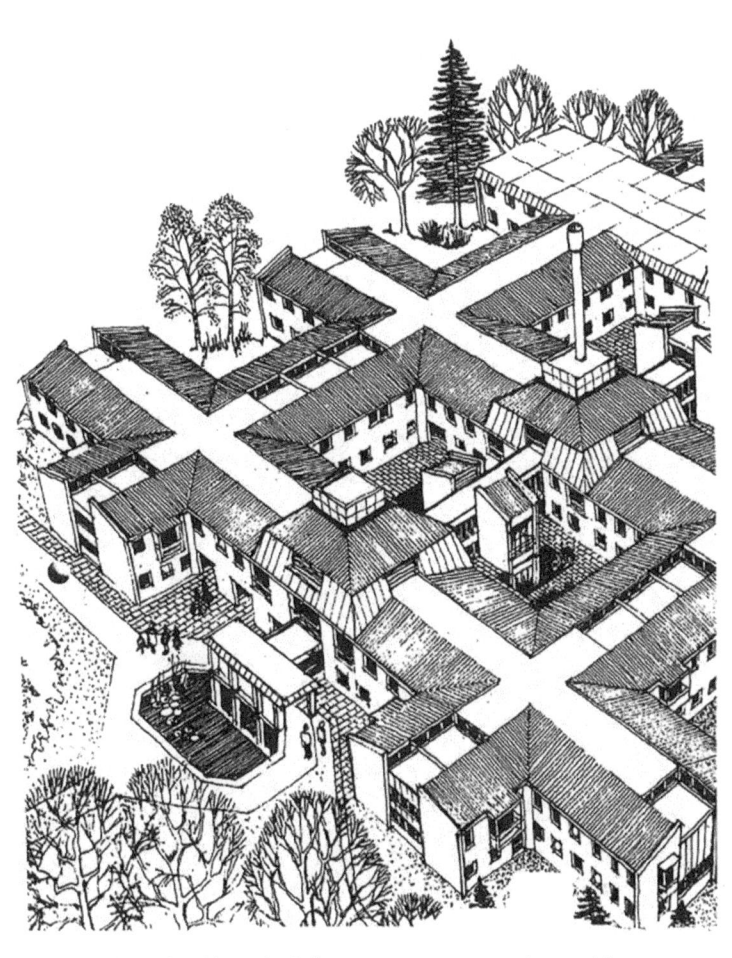

Standard hospital departments were planned in
a cruciform template – hospital Lego blocks.

ONCE UPON A TIME AROUND 1970

The last part of this chapter is intended only for readers who might be interested in understanding a little more about Nucleus hospitals and the whereabouts of some of the many built across the country. As mentioned earlier these have generally served their purpose but the best or least over developed (the purest!) should be retained until they can be replaced by smaller hospitals.

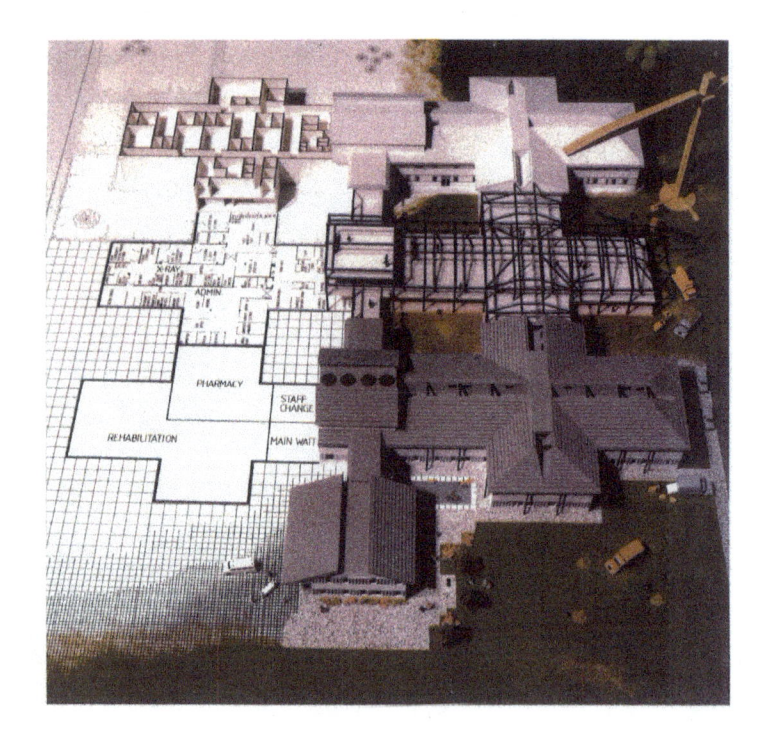

The Photograph above is of a model used to show how the Nucleus Planning and Briefing System might shape up using standard Nucleus cruciform templates.

Nucleus Hospitals that deserve a mention and possibly a visit include:

1. Maidstone Hospital – P&M Architects
2. Princess of Wales Hospital – AGP
3. Royal Bournemouth General – HLM
4. St Mary's Hospital, Newport IoW – ABK
5. Stoke City General – PTP
6. Wansbeck General – P&M

And many others, including Neath Port Talbot Hospital – SSL Architects – built this Millenium by a private finance consortium.

A visit to any of these will give the reader a feel for what was possible when teams of people were asked to design and build facilities for a uniform NHS. These Nucleus Hospitals vary in architectural interpretation which adds something unique to the design of each having all used standard data.

Interestingly, someone somehow has acquired funding of £500 million pounds to further develop/extend one of the largest Nucleus hospitals – The Royal Bournemouth General! However, those not attracting such massive investment could continue to serve a purpose with minor modifications (and even some demolition!) if existing services could be augmented by the provision of one or two smaller less extravagant state-of -the-art hospitals more relevant to today's needs but not necessarily on the same site.

Nucleus's minor downside from the use of cruciform templates ("Lego blocks") is that spaces/courtyards between two cruciform templates have often been infilled inappropriately when estate departments have been pressurised into providing more accommodation by people with little idea about its consequences.

Infills often compromise natural light, ventilation and views. Worse still, some hospitals have extended the

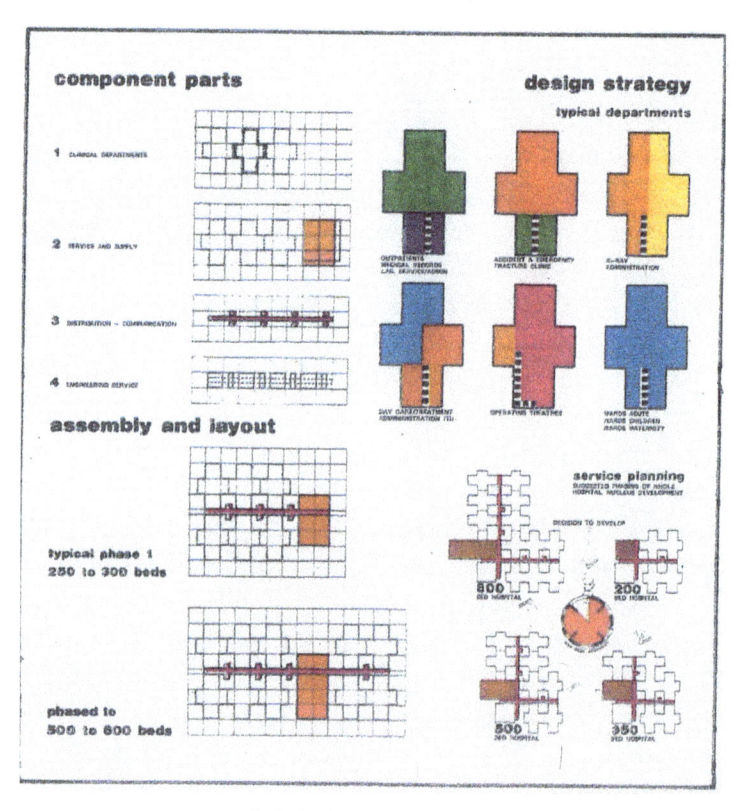

PLAN 1 (of 2) showing "Pure" Nucleus

length of the cruciform "nave" to join two cruciform templates together to form another courtyard – all too far from the maddening hospital street leading (or not leading) to confusing circulation routes.

Nucleus' major upside is that the cruciform template is changeable internally or another might be added to extend the hospital street to avoid a need for infilling. Clear guidance on how Nucleus might be extended has

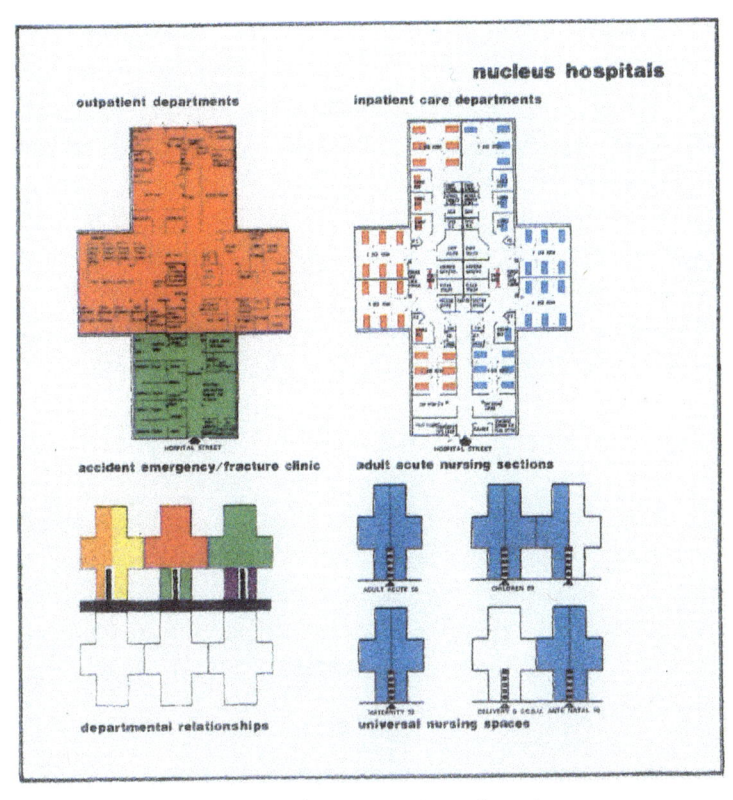

PLAN 2 (of 2) showing "Pure" Nucleus

often been ignored. The only way to deal with this is to build hospitals that cannot be extended or infilled badly by estate teams whose job is to excel at maintaining the fabric and complex engineering services. Sod's law is that the larger and more confusing a hospital gets the more likely it will become even larger and then seriously malfunction. Also, the larger a hospital gets the more difficult it becomes to replace it. It becomes part of the community patchwork and immovable.

Over the 50- year life span of Nucleus, starter hospitals for up to 300 beds with a capacity to expand have expanded and are still expanding – sometimes using any old building form other than Nucleus. Some have been modified internally (usually badly!). In the 1990's it was looking like many might reach their full potential to grow into very large hospitals of over 900 beds. This was contrary to what some of the Review Team were hoping for and would wish to discourage. They hoped Nucleus' built-in self-controlling function which had a 2 – 3 storey height restriction and an insatiable appetite for land, which was not always readily available, would kick-in. It was anticipated that, at some time soon, policy development would lead to a real contraction in the number of beds and a future need for smaller hospitals. It was becoming worrying that larger hospitals were being seen as a way of getting to grips with longer wating lists. A notion of less is more was beginning to be recognised by those that thought that the NHS had too many beds of the wrong kind.

The hospital in Neath Port Talbot was based on the usual format for a local district hospital – although the consortium did try to move it on! By its very nature and design it stands proudly as the last Nucleus hospital. When the site was purchased in 1992 it was thought that a 500-bed hospital would be needed. By 1998 the number of beds was reduced to just below 200 by accepting that other large hospitals in the vicinity should continue to take emergency and high- risk specialist referrals. When it opened in 2003 it was thought to be so much better than other recently built hospitals and was well appreciated by the local community. It is still too large especially as major acute services are elsewhere. It is in no way near the shape of things to come following Covid.

The inexperienced project team for the hospital at Neath was charged with understanding how a new hospital might improve NHS services in a locality that had a history of ill health. This was because local industries (mainly steelworks) over the decades seemed unable to consider the health and safety of their employees. A main entrance atrium was proposed to suggest a new approach to meet and greet patients to restore confidence about the services to be on offer – this was to be a good place to be and was an inspiring departure from standard Nucleus. More needs to be done by project teams when considering a hospital's place in its community and how people respond and relate to it. Its size must be a major consideration. Hospitals must be designed to help inform patients about what exactly is going on to make them feel part of the process and well again in the shortest possible time.

It was still being argued that there was a case to replace the old Neath Hospital in 1998 but given the proximity of the new site to the M4 and the string of large (Nucleus) hospitals serving South Wales along this busy motorway corridor (all worth a visit) this was the time to try something different. Unfortunately, at that time local political pressures were all consuming. Some planners felt that this was the wrong solution in 1998 – it most certainly should be in 2024.

Not many people know this but 12 Nucleus hospitals were built concurrently in Malaysia in the late 1980's - early 1990's – as a joint venture project. Six of these hospitals were provided with 314 beds and six were smaller 93 bed versions for the less populated provinces. The Malaysian government decided to go for broke – the health services were in crisis. At the same time, UK expertise was advising Iran, Hong Kong, Singapore, China and elsewhere.

Chapter 3

We will build 40 New Hospitals – but not this week

One of the earliest political promises made in 2020 when the nation was totally preoccupied with Covid was that funding would be allocated to provide the NHS with 40 new hospitals. Plans to build a new 300-bed hospital in Sutton, Surrey, were at an advanced stage and arrangements for a public consultation were in-hand. The consultation period was due to close on 1st April 2020 during the first Covid lockdown. The local NHS was allocated £500 million to invest in hospital buildings subject to this consultation.

As early as March 2020, it was looking like a proposal to build a new 300-bed hospital in Sutton based on what went before Covid might not be the best solution for the 2020s. Does it make any sense to build an old-style district general hospital, even if you call it a 'specialist emergency care hospital' in new speak, when it was becoming obvious that nucleus hospitals and other large hospitals were no longer the answer for the NHS. Everyone could see how hospitals were struggling to deal with the Covid pandemic when needing to convert wards to quadruple the number of intensive care and high-dependency beds. So much so, it was decided – wrongly – to provide never-to-be-used additional beds in open plan wards in instant temporary Nightingale hospitals – what a nightmare. Florence would have turned in her grave.

What is now clear at last is that wards with large multi-bed bays are not only unpleasant but also unmanageable. If one ever did need convincing that single rooms with ensuite toilets and showers should be the new norm it certainly should be obvious after Covid that this must be the way forward. All patients should be allowed privacy, dignity, and respect when admitted for inpatient care, especially as it is, nowadays, likely to be for a serious life-changing or life-threatening condition, if not Covid. Even if it is not as a trauma or acute admission, but to give birth or to receive care for a chronic medical or geriatric condition, surely a patient deserves to be nursed or cared for in a single room.

Having experienced Covid at its worst, it does not make sense to spend £500 million on one local NHS to build a 300-bed hospital. Less money would be better spent on new, easy, smart, smaller 2020s hospitals. Large hospitals are too big to handle. They take forever to plan and build and require updating on completion. When they facilitate bad practice, they are not easily changed and because of their size and complexity, almost impossible to replace.

From now on no hospital building should be regarded as long-life. New smaller 2020s hospitals could stand alone uncontaminated by what is going on around them if they must be built on an existing hospital site. They should be affordable, uncomplicated, understandable, flexible, intensively used, inspiring beacons of hope and promise. They should have less than 100 beds and most of these should be in single bedrooms with ensuites. These smaller hospitals should be complete and self-sufficient with all facilities in place, including emergency admissions, X-ray, theatres, recovery, out patients and rehabilitation. They would be small enough for patients, visitors and staff to be informed about what is going on within the building and promote team working with no hiding places. These smaller dynamic hospitals might look less like a hospital, with an ambience providing a more therapeutic and supportive environment. This could be instrumental in helping all users to feel informed, reassured and positive about what is on offer.

The conclusion of the public consultation in April 2020 was that the local NHS should build a 300-bed hospital in Sutton. The £500 million allocation was confirmed - of course!

Maybe a realisation that to continue to build inefficient, large hospitals is not in the interest of the NHS will only come about after a few mega hospitals have been constructed.

Large hospitals can be seen to be too much for patients and staff to comprehend when faced with a maze of rooms and corridors, which misinform, disorientate, and increase dependency. Unfortunately, some members of a lobby group called Architects for Health promote the building of European super hospitals.

Department of Health and Social Care ministers aim to have six new hospitals ready for 2025. Of the 40 on the list eight were projects already planned. The Government is committed to delivering 40 new hospitals by 2030 - as part of the biggest hospital programme in a generation.

Who knows whether the 40 new hospitals promised will fix the NHS and restore the health of the Nation? However, we should avoid building European super hospitals and large hospitals.

Chapter 4

Dear Select Committee

EVIDENCE TO THE HEALTH AND SOCIAL CARE COMMITTEE

It has been over a year since we forwarded to your committee a hard copy of our brochure[6] on 29th May 2020. In our brochure, we attempted to paint a picture of what a new, smaller, 2020 hospital might look like as a more affordable and quicker alternative to the kind of large-scale provision being proposed for Sutton, Surrey, and elsewhere. We anticipated that lessons learnt from the pandemic would expose the inadequacy of the tortuous planning processes, traditional ward and hospital layouts and highlight an urgent need to invest in new, smaller, more efficient facilities initially for trauma and elective services.

---

[6] Our brochure, *New, Easy, Fast, Smart, Smaller 2020 Hospitals to improve the NHS – after Covid-19*. Sent in hard copy to HSSC on 29th May 2020. It was subsequently circulated by your office in a digital format on 4th July 2020. This brochure was compiled during the first Coronavirus lockdown by two former employees of the Department of Health, having had access to much of the policy and health building documentation produced over many years to guide the NHS. It was thought that following Covid-19 there would be less money to invest in the replacement of the existing stock of NHS out-of-date, inflexible buildings that are no longer suitable for treating patients to modern healthcare standards.

All over the country, there is a mismatch between the quality of care skilled staff are expected to achieve using the latest equipment in the worst kind of facilities. Surgical teams urgently need an opportunity to carry out complex surgical procedures and the processes for recovery in facilities designed to reflect lessons learnt from the pandemic.

Prior to the pandemic, efforts were being made in numerous localities to save, recover, maintain, and grow existing hospitals. Large teams were planning for change to radically update or replace failing hospitals. They often produced five-year plans to implement – but here lies the problem. The pandemic has rendered such long-term plans invalid, unaffordable, and unfit for purpose.

Surely now gone are the days of long-term planning cycles and public consultations leading to gradual and begrudging ways to improve redundant hospitals or to the provision of monolithic, inflexible new hospitals. These are guaranteed to remain or become a burden for decades. Covid-19 demands that we urgently change this mind set.

We believe we are approaching a time when realistically the provision of new hospitals has to be limited by capping capital allocations for all local NHS projects. This should be seen as a positive policy. A way to achieve this would be to inform local NHSs that they can bid to build a new, smaller 2020s trauma or elective hospital of up to 10,000 sq. m. if they can demonstrate that this would foster a radical new approach to their service provision, including, if possible, at an alternative location to the existing hospital. Existing hospitals were probably built in the right place for the 1900s but are most likely to be in the wrong place for the 2020s. A strategy providing a network of smaller hospitals would make land acquisition easier.

There is just not enough capacity in the NHS to deal with the current backlog in the short- and medium-term, so a rapid construction programme should always be a condition of funding. We are imagining the production of brand-new, smaller hospitals to kick-start a revitalised hospital construction programme. Stockpiles of data and guidance exist to inform how new, smaller hospitals might be planned, designed and commissioned in the 2020s. Example solutions used in our brochure were based on this wealth of information to suggest how (A) a trauma centre and (B) an elective centre might be planned to create new, smaller 2020 hospitals within a locality to save a need to, recover, maintain, and grow existing hospitals.

The pandemic has shown that we can learn to move quickly to provide the NHS with equipment and temporary facilities staff demanded for their own hospitals (they did not want to use those over-sized, wasteful and nightmarish Nightingale hospitals). It has also shown that new and better facilities are urgently required to tackle the waiting lists that are a consequence of the pandemic and that these should build in measures to contain Covid-19 surges.

To summarise, a new smaller hospital in the right location should probably be sited away from, but used in conjunction with, an existing hospital, be assembled quickly, be affordable within a fixed capital cost (up to 10,000 sq. m. in size), and have more relevance to the way surgical teams will have to work in the future. It should also be uncomplicated, patient friendly, therapeutic, flexible, and intensively used.

Now is the time to showcase how adaptable, new, smaller hospitals can be provided quickly to replace our many failing hospitals. These would lift morale, renew confidence, and house and promote even better services throughout the NHS. The primary aim should be to demonstrate that the NHS will require less beds, not more, through improved performances in the right kind of facilities in the aftermath of this life changing pandemic.

If your committee really is interested in recognising how much the NHS estate and existing hospital buildings are straightjacketing innovation as services need to evolve to meet emerging challenges, here is a tentative road map:

1. DHSC to appoint a control team to set up parameters for a network of new, smaller 2020s hospitals and project manage the provision and evaluation of the first wave.
2. Organise an open invitation to local NHSs with a five-year plan, asking them to put their plans on the back burner and, instead, apply to be selected to build a new, smaller 2020s trauma or elective hospital.
3. Set up a selection process for a first wave network focussing on the following: the applicant's surgical team's performance and their proposals to deal

with waiting lists; management and staff cohesion; an ability to show how they might operate the new facility; their ways and means of demonstrating a better performance from new facilities; availability of a potential site and its location; how each local NHS is ready to move quickly to provide a new facility, and, on completion, how the evacuation of existing hospital accommodation might be used to improve other priority services including long Covid.
4. Completion, commissioning and a fully operational service should be documented as a case study for a second wave.
5. Each new smaller hospital should be evaluated to report on performance.

We are looking for no more than an indication that some of our suggestions might be relevant to a rebuilt NHS, taking account of Covid-19 and the need for an increased capacity to deal with the backlog. Also, we are looking for signs that your committee is taking seriously a need to build the right kind of hospitals to support the future work of the NHS and care services. Buildings cannot put more staff in place to deal with the backlog but they can give staff within the NHS better facilities to help improve and increase performances.

LB and RG

3rd September 2021

Chapter 5

Dear Secretary of State

Department of Health and Social Care London

14th September 2022

Dear Secretary of State

An outline blueprint for the NHS (which has been staring us in the face!)

We are not even sure you will ever get to see/read this but...!

We believe someone in your office should see/read this letter and study its attachments, which we have peddled around since soon after the Covid outbreak in 2020. These attachments form an outline blueprint that follows on from decades of work undertaken by your predecessors and numerous people at the department at great expense to the taxpayer. It is only now that its relevance to the current difficulties facing the NHS has become clear. It is too difficult a concept to be carried forward by the NHS and can only be actioned by your department. Hopefully someone will see how this kind of blueprint could compliment the rollout of the 160 community diagnostic centres being set up to diagnose patients quickly. This recent initiative needs the back-up of a progressive hospital service.

You will need to shortcut the cumbersome process currently in place to procure hospital buildings on an ad hoc basis which looks to reinvent the wheel for every project. It is time for your department to take control of this process and face up to the obvious need to provide the NHS with new healthcare facilities quickly starting with trauma and elective care specialities. The NHS's inadequate stock of existing hospital buildings is a major obstacle to a much-needed change of strategy.

This outline blueprint was included in our 'Evidence to the Health and Social Care Committee', dated 3rd September 2021. This suggested that the design of new hospitals has a direct bearing on how the NHS might recover from its own trauma, cope with the vaccine-shackled virus from now on, and get to grips with the massive backlog caused by the pandemic. Perhaps not unreasonably, the committee's interest was restrained – it was an exceptionally busy time and the issue of resource allocation in healthcare is perhaps too complex.

Also, you will see from our attachments that we tried to engage with the Epsom and St Helier University Hospitals NHS Trust re. a new hospital at Sutton (our brochure) and St George's University Hospital re. a new trauma centre. These approaches, as expected, were unsuccessful – clearly it is easier to ignore the substantial changes now needed to improve the NHS after the pandemic and to limp on doing what went before. This is the crux of the matter!

We do not need to hear back from you. This outline blueprint and its intellectual property belongs to your department. We are now almost too old and exhausted to care and have done our bit! We just wish that someone could just get on with using this or something like it for the sake of the NHS and the people waiting to be treated and provided with a responsive service.

Now is the time to stop planning those too few, redundant large/mega hospitals and to get on with fixing the NHS by building many smaller, smarter, hospitals quickly in the right place...

Yours sincerely

LB and RG

Dear Secretary of State did not get in touch – not even an acknowledgement from her Private Office – ships had passed in the night! This secretary of state was reshuffled to another berth in Mr Sunak's first cabinet which seems hardly surprising. Also, no one in their right mind would expect that the replacement would delve into the pending tray of a short-lived predecessor. This provoked the thought to write the first 'Dear Susan...' paperback.

A second secretary of state was sent a complimentary copy of the first 'Dear Susan...' paperback as soon as it was published - on 13th July 2023. Again, no acknowledgement from his private office.

A third secretary of state was appointed on 13th November 2023 in another cabinet reshuffle. A complimentary copy of the first 'Dear Susan...' paperback was sent immediately to her office to welcome her to her new job. It was likely to be binned by her private office – but maybe there was an outside chance that this secretary of state might dip into it before the next reshuffle!

Perhaps no secretary of state or their numerous support staff would think that there could be a decorator/patient/retired hospital architect and Rosemary out there who might be able to suggest using what had gone before to lever out a blueprint from the wealth of published guidance. A blueprint that might work today following the Covid-19 pandemic.

In a nutshell, NHS staff have the skills needed and there are probably enough of them trained up and ready to start all over again - even though they may feel they have had enough. However, most of the time they have the wrong vehicle to change speed, break new ground and to help drive forward a new strategy.

Chapter 6

Enough is really Enough

It is easy to believe that nowadays admission to the NHS for treatment is nothing but a lottery. Some win and some lose. Clearly there can be no guarantees given for treating injuries or ill health but much more could be done to encourage organisational competence in buildings that are fit for purpose.

If hospital buildings transmit a feeling of obsolescence and neglect by the way they are planned and by looking badly maintained it will affect staff motivations, morale, patients' confidence, and often get in the way of treatment and a timely recovery. In some hospitals it is difficult not to want to be discharged soon after you are admitted because a downward spiral of unwellness and helplessness overcomes you in addition to what is expected after a surgical or medical procedure. A concern for patients' privacy, better meals, cleaner wards, with nurses and other staff more able to be alert to a patients' needs would all improve the patients' experience. These improvements must go hand in hand with a therapeutic approach to care and treatment in efficiently run facilities where patients can feel confident about what ls happening to them and why.

The aim should be to reduce admissions to as short a period as possible. This can be helped by providing hospitals that meet improved standards not far short of what one would expect from a good hotel. Better hospitals with the latest no-expense-spared equipment could help increase the turnover of patients using staff already in the NHS and help improve outcomes. Hospitals should be built to help save lives.

> *Everything about the NHS is too big to handle. It is time to downsize and for all users to feel part of something that is tangible. To help achieve this, there surely can be nothing better than to build new, easy, smart, smaller hospitals quickly so that 'enough' becomes 'really enough' and confidence in the NHS can be restored.*

As of January 2024, 7.5 million people were waiting on the NHS for a surgical or medical procedure.

'Public satisfaction with the NHS has slumped to its lowest level ever recorded. Just 29% said they were satisfied with the NHS in 2022 with waiting times and staff shortages the biggest concerns' – British Social Attitudes Survey, 29th March 2023.

So, what might this "hotel" look like and how might bedrooms be arranged to make a hospital feel less like a hospital?

Chapter 7 describes how bedrooms might be provided in 32 bedroom 'wards' sub-divided into two 16 bedroom 'sub-wards' or four 8 bedroom clusters. Plans 3 and 4 show how this might be achieved for example:

DEAR SUSAN... WE'RE ALL GOING ON A SUMMER HOLIDAY...

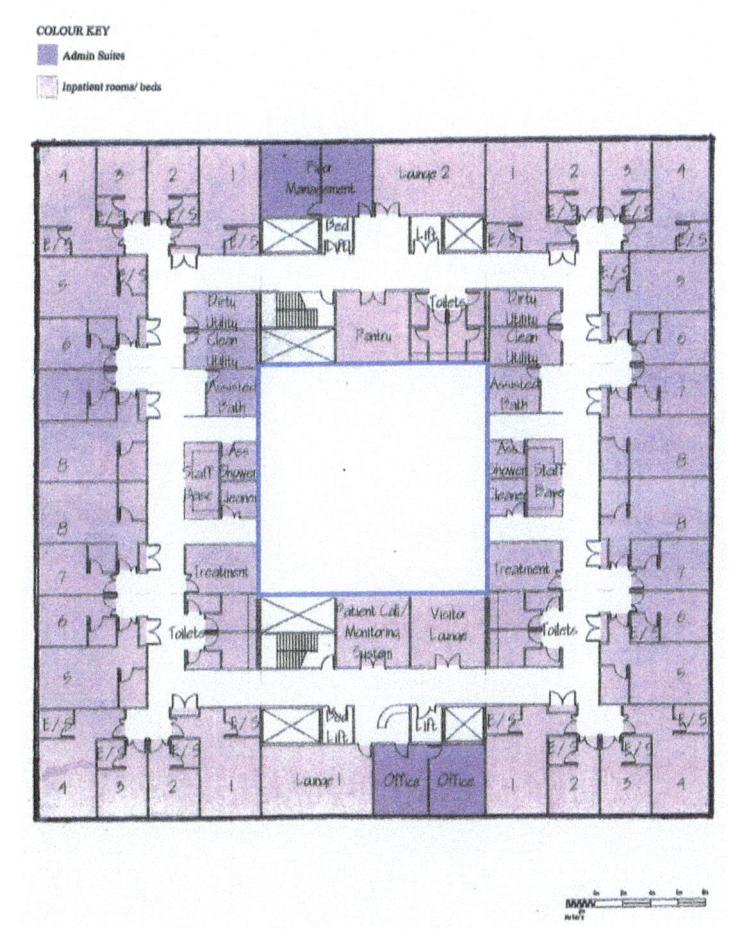

PLAN 3 showing a 32 bedroom 'ward'.

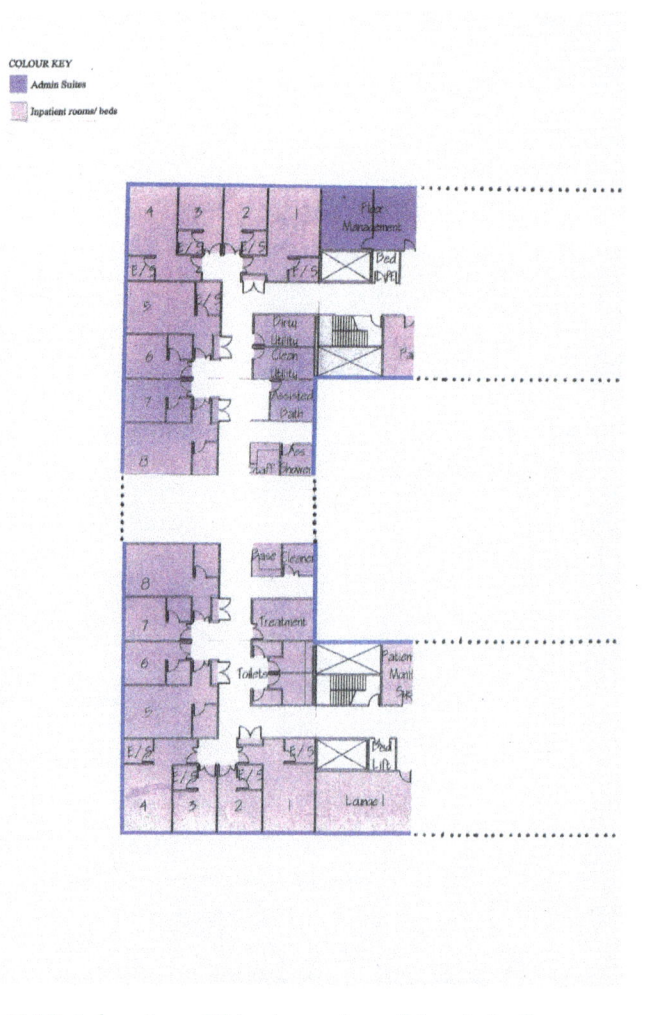

PLAN 4 showing a 32 bedroom 'ward' "exploded"
into two 16 bedroom 'sub-wards' and
four 8 bedroom clusters

DEAR SUSAN... WE'RE ALL GOING ON A SUMMER HOLIDAY...

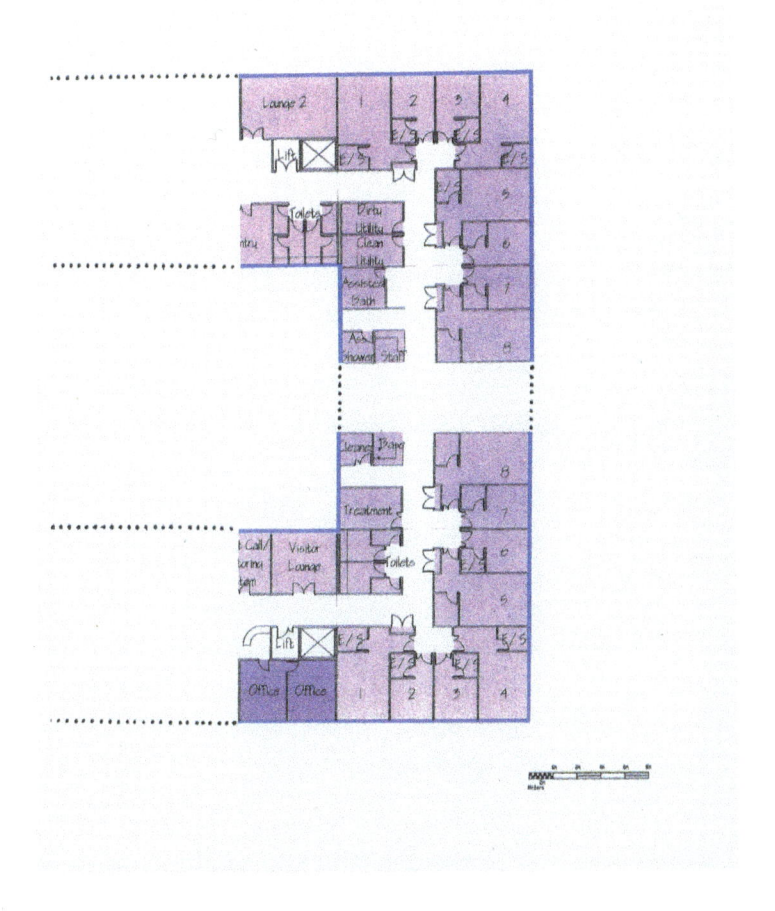

A 32 bedroom 'ward'

This 32 bedroom 'ward' is divided into four by eight-bedroom clusters. These might be allocated for specialist treatment groups, high dependency patients, medium dependency 'step down,' or women only, men only, children, older people, or allocated randomly.

It has a mix of single and double bedrooms each with an ensuite. The double bedrooms are to allow a spouse/partner/carer to stay with an adult patient needing assistance or a parent to stay with an unwell child or to allow a patient needing a longer length of stay to have a 'place like home'!

Each 16 bedroom 'sub ward' has a lounge, a nursing station and a treatment room. The 32 bedroom 'ward' has a patient monitoring room, visitors lounge and a pantry to distribute an appetising choice of meals.

Chapter 7

Non – Fantasy Smaller Hospitals

After the worst of Covid, the NHS now must deal with a constant flow of emergencies and a massive backlog of less urgent but significant injuries and illnesses that are crippling the population. A new strategy is required. This could provide a rapidly built new generation of major trauma centres and elective care centres. Also, it could provide a range of other rapidly built centres like those for accident and emergency, women and children, chronic care, elderly care, rehabilitation, cancer care, renal centres, and so on, in new, fast, easy, smart, smaller, hospitals. However, the immediate need is for trauma and elective care surgical centres. These can be built to sidestep what went before and what is going on now to inappropriately transform larger, failing, older hospitals, many of which are of the wrong time and are now in the wrong place. All specialties other than trauma and elective day care could continue to use suitable and better maintained existing hospitals like the last generation of nucleus hospitals until they also need replacing with new smaller hospitals.

What would a network of new, easy, fast, smart, smaller, hospitals all have in common given that, for example, major trauma centres and elective care centres are in many ways quite a different beast? Also, some way

NON – FANTASY SMALLER HOSPITALS

down the line it might also be necessary to build new smaller hospitals for other specialties.

Non - Fantasy smaller hospitals should be:

- Able to be built quickly.
- Built and equipped to stand-alone, located where they are needed
- Uncomplicated, understandable, and flexible.
- No larger than 10,000 square metres.
- No higher than 4 stories high.
- Should have standardized/interchangeable suites, e.g., theatre suite, X-ray suite, etc.
- Smaller than 100 bedrooms (max) for an inpatient hospital – provided with mostly single and double bedrooms all with ensuites, except in ITU.
- More like a hotel than a hospital.
- Accessible to air and road ambulances.
- Not able to be extended.
- Replaced when they become obsolete and as soon as someone thinks of extending them badly.
- Therapeutic and inspire confidence.
- Able to provide free and accessible parking.
- Accessible by rail and good public transport.

The above criteria could fit both trauma care and elective care, and many other specialties.

The major trauma centre would be 'open all hours' and could be fully planned and equipped with suites for emergency triage, X-ray, two or four theatre suites plus recovery and intensive care, rehabilitation, consultation/orthoplastic clinic, i.e., be totally self-sufficient for treating trauma and for the long road to recovery. It would have mostly single bedrooms with ensuites except in recovery or intensive care spaces. It would have 64 bedrooms (max) in two 'wards'. The 32-bedroom 'wards' could be divided into two 16 bedroom 'sub-wards' or four eight-bedroom clusters. These eight-room clusters might be allocated for high and medium dependency or women only, men only, children, older people, specialist treatment groups, or allocated randomly. It could be that a mix of single and double bedrooms might be provided to allow a spouse/partner/carer to stay with an adult patient who is needing their assistance or a parent to stay with an unwell child. Surely not too much to ask of an efficient future health service aiming to reduce how long a patient needs to stay.

Major trauma centres might be located not necessarily on existing hospital sites but where they are needed, say around the M25 or along other motorways connected by air ambulance and fast road ambulance services with a mainline railway station within spitting distance.

The elective care centre, being a day-care facility, would be 'open from 7am 'til midnight'. It too would be fully planned and equipped with suites for reception, X-ray, more theatres and recovery suites than an inpatient hospital as beds will not be needed, comfortable lounges for second stage recovery, rehabilitation, consultation/clinics. This too would be totally self-sufficient for day-care procedures.

Elective care centres could be located alongside trauma centres or be sited to be more accessible for local communities if necessary on an existing hospital site but self-contained and to stand alone to be managed separately from the existing hospital. Elective care centres should be

NON — FANTASY SMALLER HOSPITALS

accessible to air ambulances as well as road ambulances and public transport.

A network of non - fantasy smaller hospitals should have linked communications to manage movement of staff, supplies, and patient admissions.

LB hoped that by the time he retired every hospital would be fit for purpose. He thought that at some time in the not-too-distant future the NHS would need fewer beds in smaller hospitals. These would be bright, shiny, optimistic, and therapeutic machines for healing which are full of hope and promise. Less staff would be doing so much more to mend/cure any condition/symptom and reduce the need for lengthy hospital admissions. A quick turnround of patients and a community support network with direct communication to these smaller hospitals would put right without fuss any mishap on the journey to a long and fit life.

Fantasy or wishful thinking maybe, but the Covid-19 pandemic has left an opportunity to change things using much of what is already available and already in place in the NHS. A touch on the rudder is needed to quickly straighten things out and to stop the NHS from going round and round in circles.

Nucleus hospitals now are a thing of the past. At that time some people thought they were too prescriptive, and many found its level of standardisation difficult, preferring a bespoke solution for each service. They argued that standardisation stifled creativity on individual schemes. Sadly, some of these individual schemes had square wheels. Nucleus met many of its challenges but on looking back it maybe was too big a hammer to crack a nut.

In 1975, when promoting nucleus hospitals, the health minister said, 'The NHS had in many areas not achieved the benefits from being a centralised service.' Maybe in the 2020s it might be appropriate to argue again for an element of standardisation so that the two key areas of need might be met by providing new, fast, smarter, smaller, hospitals using the latest technology for trauma care and elective care based on the criteria set out above. This might get the bull/NHS by the horns, leaving all other services to creatively determine how they use all existing hospitals needing an upgrade until they too feel a need to get on a smaller hospital bandwagon. We are talking here about a new start in providing efficient facilities for surgery to alleviate the pain and discomfort of so many people – and quickly.

Enough could be much more – someone should get on with it! Are there no longer lively clever Under-Secretaries in the Department of Health and Social Care or somewhere else in the Civil Service like the Treasury to tell their political masters and their advisors to stop sitting on their hands? They should be looking for medium-term strategies that can start to be delivered quickly to get the NHS out of its deep hole and deal with the nation's health issues.

Non-Fantasy 'wards' of 32 single and double bedrooms – surely not?

In 1977 the 'pure' Nucleus cruciform template was planned to provide 56 beds in two 28 bed wards – see PLAN 2. Each 28-bed ward had four six bed bays and four single rooms.

NON – FANTASY SMALLER HOSPITALS

In 1990 the cruciform template was increased in area and replanned to provide 48 beds in two 24 bed wards. Each 24-bed ward had three larger six bed bays and six single rooms.

Just imagine the lengthy discussions about nursing practices and the cost implications for the NHS that accompanied this change. Some believed that this would inevitably lead to larger hospitals, increased staffing ratios and unaffordable costs. Others thought that this should help reduce the number of beds required and encourage a shorter length of stay in hospital for many acute and chronic conditions.

So why do we need more single rooms and what is wrong with sharing multi-bed bays/rooms?

LB's experience is that the NHS and its patients deserve better. It is difficult to gauge just how much out of date, drab, crowded, uncomfortable, too busy and noisy multi-bed bays affect patient outcomes and staff morale – who has time to care? However positive you are about your condition, it soon becomes clear that it is likely to worsen the longer you remain anchored to your bed or chair in a cubicle with a lack of space around the bed in which it is impossible to sleep, be washed and toileted or to have cleaned around orthopaedic equipment. Home begins to feel as if it might provide a perfect aid to daily living and recovery because of its familiarity, close travel distances, meal preferences, and your life is in your hands.

If you cannot be allowed home to get better, why not allow patients to recover in a hospital more like an hotel?

Chapter 8

A Healthier Population

One thing is for sure – no matter how good or bad the NHS is we are all going to die soon enough - somehow!. Maybe the NHS serves its purpose exactly as it is/seems by doing its best to assist us all with a way out of this world. Is its purpose/role less about fixing and more about preparing? It could be that this is well understood and is why the country so supportively and repeatedly clapped the NHS and painted rainbows during Covid.

So, does anything need changing?

Of-course it does – so why not start with providing an effective NHS for all those requiring either Trauma Care or Elective Day Care in highly efficient smaller hospitals? This could have a real impact on what can/should/must be done to achieve a healthier population but is this all too simple?

LB believes there is a need for change/action but clearly has been unsuccessful in getting his message across. So here is his last roll of the dice even though the first 'Dear Susan…' was not worth acknowledging and certainly not worth reading by a target audience that seemingly did not understand its message.

Imagine, new, easy, fast, smart, smaller hospitals proliferating across the country located where it makes sense and linked to/networked by clever communication systems, air and road ambulances for patient and staff movements and with drones, white van man and Amazon delivering supplies. Also, imagine providing a first wave of Trauma Care and Elective Day Care hospitals, able to deal with anything thrown at them like a sophisticated "MASH" emergency field hospital as depicted in the TV series and in film. Surely not a difficult concept? Can you also imagine staff being fully informed because of the reduced scale of the hospital, in complete control of clinical outcomes, enthusiastically working as a team in the right context to get our unwell population back on its feet again? Plus an added bonus that hospital buildings could be beautiful, therapeutic and uplifting for patients, staff and visitors. These should be places you want to be in if you have something wrong with you, in the community they should serve well. Can this ever be made to happen in the real world of the NHS?.

Of-course it can. So, what might a smaller hospital look like?.

PLAN 5 shows a starter Nucleus hospital providing up to 275 beds. You may recall from Chapter 2 that standard hospital departments were planned in cruciform templates – hospital Lego blocks. Plan 5 also shows how it could eventually provide 800 beds or more in a phased development.

PLAN 6 shows (a blueprint for the NHS?) the shape of a new Trauma Centre (with inpatient bedrooms) or an Elective Day Care Centre (with no bedrooms but more operating theatres and recovery lounges) in a non-cruciform arrangement.

By comparing these two plans, the downsizing to arrive at the critical mass for a smaller hospital might be more easily understood. Plan 5 shows how Nucleus could be expanded from a starter hospital into a too large "mega" hospital. In its new downsize form in Plan 6 it cannot (and should not) be expanded. Once built it should remain a new, easy, fast, smart, smaller hospital.

Please apply yourselves. These plans could not be any simpler. They are included because the word game played in the first 'Dear Susan...' paperback deliberately avoided using illustrations and plans and this seems not to have worked. Hopefully a sight of these plans and those in Chapter 9 will not provide readers with an excuse to turn a blind eye and to pull the wool over it!

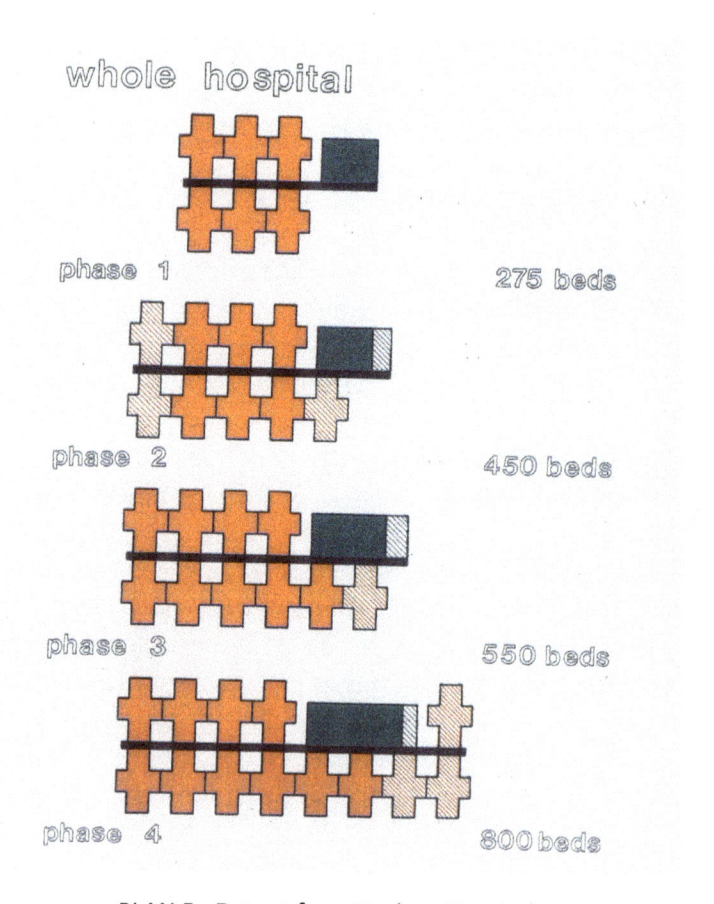

PLAN 5 - Extract from Nucleus Hospital
Planning Aid – November 1975

Nucleus was low rise, usually two storeys high and up to three storeys on a sloping site. It was capable of being phased, easily extended and when necessary enlarged to be updated.

DEAR SUSAN... WE'RE ALL GOING ON A SUMMER HOLIDAY...

- What next after Covid?   3

- Why not smaller hospitals?   2

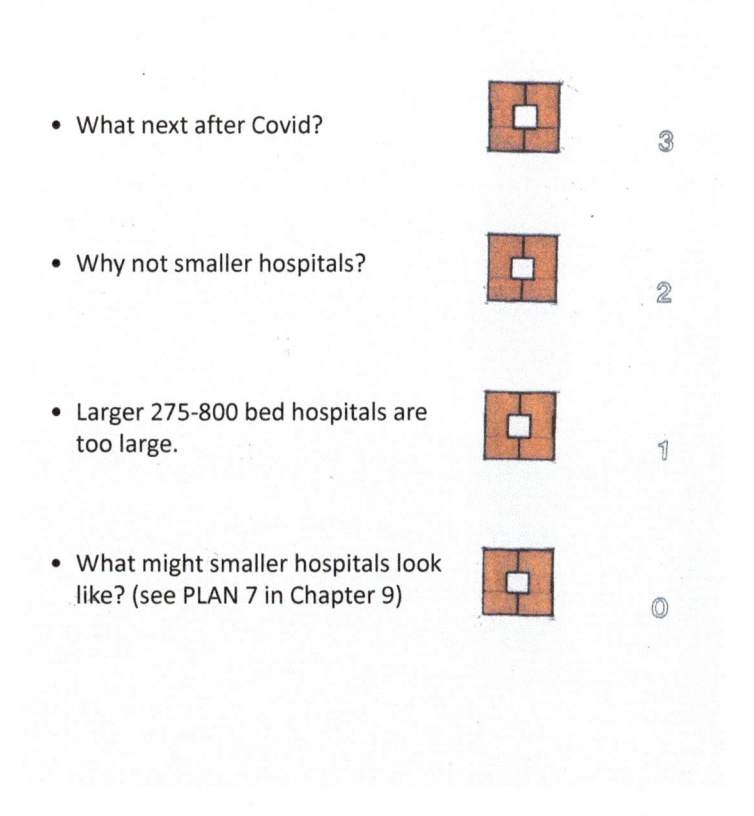

- Larger 275-800 bed hospitals are too large.   1

- What might smaller hospitals look like? (see PLAN 7 in Chapter 9)   0

PLAN 6 - This is set beside PLAN 5 to compare a smaller hospital with original Nucleus. It shows how a four storey Trauma Centre and an Elective Day Care Centre might be sized using Nucleus data.

If you are at all interested in looking inside an orange Nucleus cruciform template illustrated in PLAN 5 above, please refer back to PLAN 2 on page 23 in Chapter 2 showing 'Pure' Nucleus.

Likewise, for an example as to how an orange square with a square hole shown above in PLAN 6 above might be planned/fitted-out, see PLAN 3 on page 43 in Chapter 6 which shows a 32 bedroom 'ward'.

PLAN 7, pages 62&63 in Chapter 9 should also be referred to if you wish to see in more detail how layouts might shape up for treatment suites in non- fantasy Trauma Care and Elective Care Centres.

Now rest your heads for now!

Chapter 9

Why so B..... Persistent?

As described in the first 'Dear Susan...' paperback, there is nothing better than a pandemic and admission to a large teaching hospital to make you believe that there is a need for change - but who will listen?.

So, how come LB still thinks he has some of the answers?

It is because LB was there when something huge was happening. Not 'Once Upon a Time in 1970' but certainly in the early 1990's when he was asked to review the previous 20 years of Nucleus guidance. Also, to find a way of updating the Nucleus Briefing and Design System and the hospital building programme short term. LB was also to see if there was a way forward for Nucleus long term and whether it should it be re-configured, replaced or aborted.

Its replacement was anticipated by some of those familiar with the project with a real conviction about where it should be heading in future. Nucleus had hundreds of contributors and believers - many of who are now kicking up the daisies and no longer have a voice about our floundering NHS. It was some of those believers who foresaw a significant shift in strategy in the provision of hospital buildings well before Covid.

As mentioned earlier, this sequel now includes plans to illustrate smaller hospitals. LB now fully accepts that his words fail or fall on cloth ears but that someone out there might pause over an illustration or two.

PLAN 7 is included for those who would like to see more substance. Looking at this is not compulsory – hopefully it will not mislead. This shows how the same building envelope/box/or container might be used for both new, easy, fast, smart, smaller Trauma Care Centres 'open all hours" and Elective Care Day Care Centres 'open from 7am 'til midnight' – or for any other speciality like Renal Care (also see description in Chapter7).

It is thought that this four-storey form could accommodate any speciality. This could be arranged by choosing from a selection of suites. Try to envisage a choice of assembly – like choosing options/specifications for a new car – interesting for some!

PLANS 8 and 9 are a bit of fun to show how three types of smaller hospitals might be located/sited on a couple of real existing hospital sites.

Now flip back to Chapter 7 – Is the description of Non-Fantasy Hospitals helped by the plans included in this 'Dear Susan...' sequel?

If not, it is time for LB to put his best foot forward and enjoy retirement on holiday swimming to and from his harbour wall in Greece. This is fine when you are well in to retirement but come on! – there is so much needing to be done by those in a position to achieve change unless they are expecting that the NHS can transform itself.

WHY SO B..... PERSISTENT?

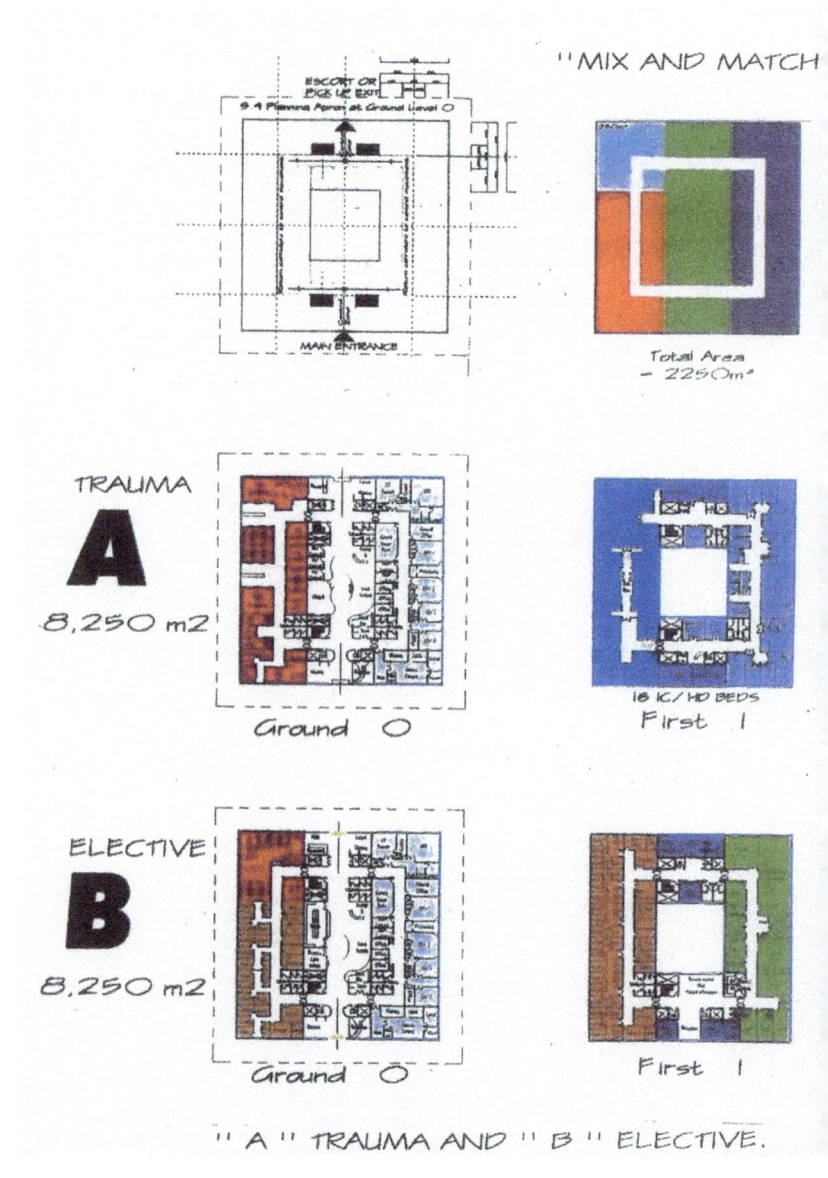

PLAN 7 Non – Fantasy Smaller Hospitals

DEAR SUSAN... WE'RE ALL GOING ON A SUMMER HOLIDAY...

SUITES OF ACCOMMODATION

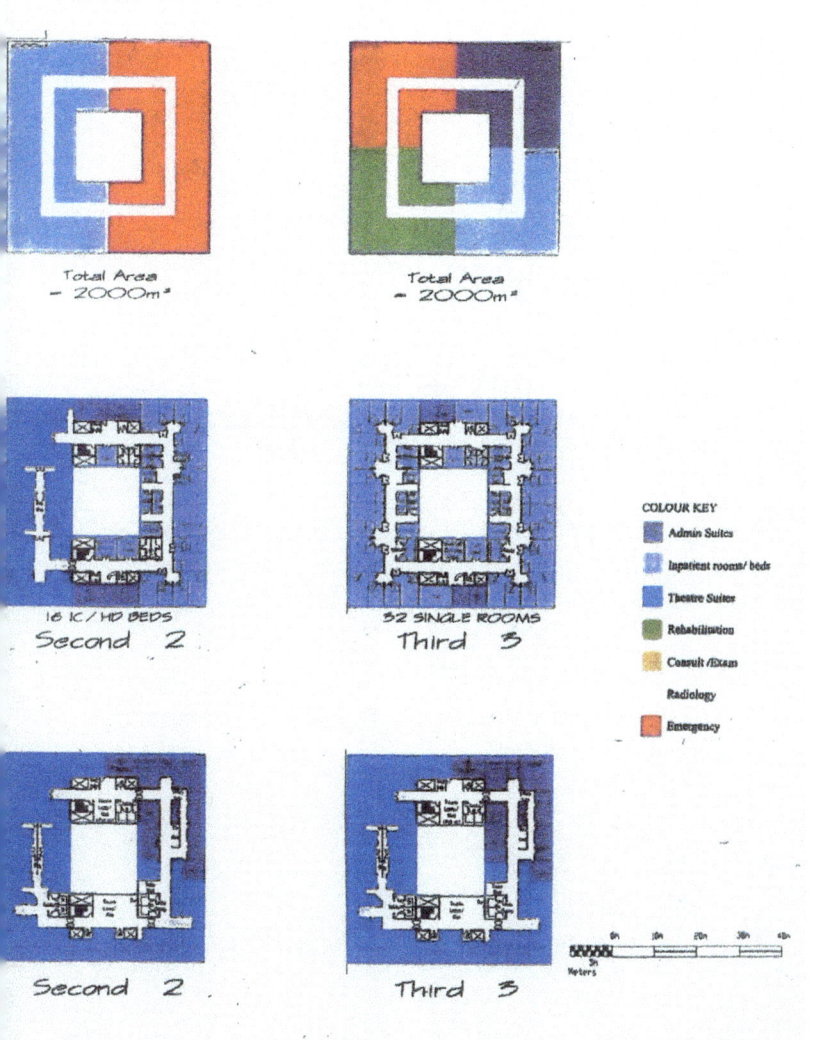

Total Area ~ 2000m²

Total Area ~ 2000m²

16 IC/HD BEDS
Second 2

32 SINGLE ROOMS
Third 3

COLOUR KEY
- Admin Suites
- Inpatient rooms/ beds
- Theatre Suites
- Rehabilitation
- Consult /Exam
- Radiology
- Emergency

Second 2

Third 3

63

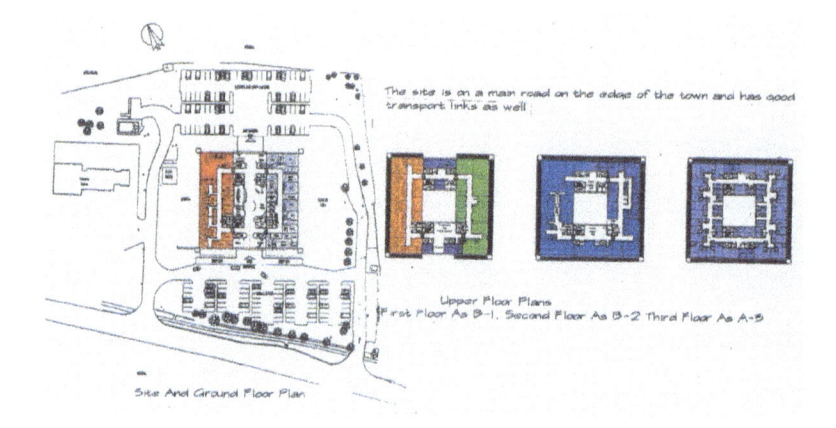

PLAN 8 Non – Fantasy Smaller Hospitals

Do these non – fantasy smaller hospitals all have to be in square boxes?

No! They can be of any shape you care to think up as long as they work but they should stand alone, not be extendable and fit the criterion set out in Chapter 7.

Also, they should be inspiring beacons of hope for the NHS and all those people needing timely healthcare.

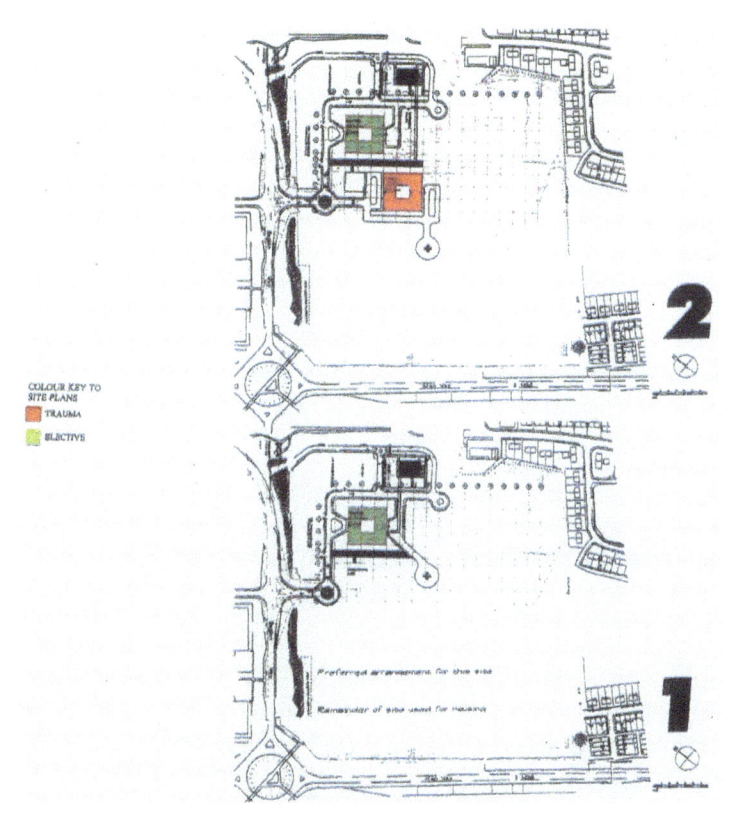

PLAN 9 Non – Fantasy Smaller Hospitals

Major Trauma Centres should be located where they are needed and not necessarily on an existing hospital site. Elective Care Centres could be located alongside trauma centres or be sited to be more accessible to local communities if necessary on an existing hospital site – see Chapter 7.

A louder voice than LB's is needed to argue the case for a buildings' led initiative for the NHS to provide smaller hospitals. It is highly unlikely to come from the Architectural profession. Most architects usually have to wait to be asked and are then expected to do as they are briefed. There are some architectural practices who are bursting to design a high-tech futures hospital. Some, when leading their field internationally, have never been commissioned to design a relevant ground breaking health care building for the NHS (like Rogers, Foster, Hadid and Grimshaw). What a difference these and some of the bright, younger practices might make, given half a chance.

With the challenge set out in this sequel, they might join a control group of interested and committed health care professionals in providing a network of smaller hospitals and look beyond the traditional mindset for the procurement of hospital buildings. This might help the NHS to make a massive leap forward and to get on with what it does best in looking after the health of the nation.

Chapter 10

Epilogue according to LB

Does it all end here - not quite!

"**NHS waiting list could top eight million by next summer, even if doctor strikes cease, according to modelling work carried out by The Health Foundation charity**" – October 2023.

An extract from the first 'Dear Susan…' paperback 'Introduction' is worth another shout from a mountain top!

"LB hoped that, by the time he retired, every hospital would be fit for purpose. He expected that at some time in the not-too-distant-future fewer large hospitals would be needed. These would be replaced by bright, shiny, optimistic and therapeutic smaller hospitals with less staff doing so much more to mend/cure any condition/symptom to reduce the need for lengthy hospital admissions and invasive treatments – with many diagnose and minor treatments being sorted online to bypass a failing GP service. Waiting lists would be a thing of the past – A responsive NHS."

"Perhaps this was all wishful thinking faced with a Covid pandemic but LB's 'shock horror' experience

EPILOGUE ACCORDING TO LB

from being referred to St George's confirmed the reality that the NHS was nowhere providing the right kind of hospitals needed for the 2020's and the massive backlog caused mainly by Covid could not be resolved without a drastic change of government policy".

The NHS cannot change magically but could improve its performance with the help of the Target Audience listed in Chapter 1. Having been sent a complimentary copy of the first 'Dear Susan...' paperback most of them appear to be uncontactable, disinterested or they went awol/missing while on holiday. Maybe this is as it should be having been bombarded with a blueprint for the NHS out of the blue! However, perhaps they could also spend more time looking as if they are doing something about the health of the nation by providing the NHS with "transformative solutions and supportive vital well- resourced working environments"[7] – in much better smaller hospitals.

---

[7] BBCs' Michelle Roberts, on 27th October 2023, quoted the President of the Royal College of Surgeons – England as follows:

"To tackle waiting lists in a meaningful and sustainable way, we need transformative solutions"

"Crucially we must improve staff morale and retention. The Government's commitment to grow the healthcare workforce is welcome. However, recruiting new staff is only half the solution. Providing a supportive, well-resourced working environment is vital"

Attempts by LB in November 2023 to clarify exactly what a "supportive, well-resourced working environment" is and why it is "vital" failed miserably having sent a complimentary copy of the first 'Dear Susan...' to Mr President on 31st October – clearly silence is golden or is it?

Acknowledgement and Epitaph (Revised)

To all multidisciplinary teams who worked on the Nucleus Hospital Building Programme which was the purple patch of NHS Design Guidance for three decades. This data is still used as a benchmark. It was always intended to be used to promote change and innovation. All the many people involved thought that national guidelines were crucial for a better and fairer NHS.

Also, thanks to the late:

Howard Goodman

Percy Ward

Ceri Davies

Brian Hitchcox

Under Secretary 1984

Sheila Scott

Phillip Powell

Peter Skinner

Richard Burton

David Hutchinson

Danuta Blasczczyk

ACKNOWLEDGEMENT AND EPITAPH (REVISED)

Jane Lamb

Tony Jones

Ron Graham

Natalie Slier

Maurice Fillery

And the not so late:

Minister of State for Health 1975

Mike Meager

Geof Mayers

Mike Singh

Don Eastwood

John Hall

John Meek

Bill Simpson

Jonathan Millman

Stuart Robinson

Simon Mills

Judy Nolan (McTaggart)

Colin Gillert

Mungo Smith

Justin De Syllas

Ian Simpson

Derek Acton Stowe

Chris Paulley

Ian Wells

Robert Scott

Robin Beynon

The great and the good who pioneered the R&D work for "Best Buy" and "Harness" hospitals and all that went before Nucleus under William Tatton Brown.

The St George's major trauma team

The St George's Chief Transformation Officer

St George's X-Ray department

The Chair of St George's, Epsom and St Helier NHS Health Group

District and GP practice nurses

The chairman of the Parliamentary Health and Social Care Committee 2020-2022

The family WhatsApp Group

Niece Beryl who merged the two 'Dear Susan...' documents.

And last but not least – Dear Susan

The reader that gets this far will see from the "Epitaph" that too many NHS enthusiasts are no longer with us, so their contributions are mainly historical although LB hopes he has represented them well.

However, one former Chief Architect to the Department of Health is still standing. He was sent a copy of the first "Dear Susan …" paperback and it seems reasonable to include his thoughts.

> Dear L and R
>
> Thank you for the copy of your paperback "Dear Susan …" I read it eagerly and felt your frustration. Nobody is really listening these days in spite of the carbon copy crises we experience like the recovery from WW2 and again in the aftermath of the Oil Crisis in the 70's. Here we are again.
>
> I was fascinated by a radio programme this week which made the observation that the Japanese economic recovery after WW2 was led by their architects, especially Kenso Tange (one of my heroes).
>
> ....
>
> Hey ho.
>
> Keep in touch
>
> G
>
> 18th January 2024

The dotted line above represents a helpful reality check from G about the fore runners to Nucleus – well before LB's time!.

Unfortunately, Kenso Tange has passed away so another good idea bites the dust!

Another Last Word

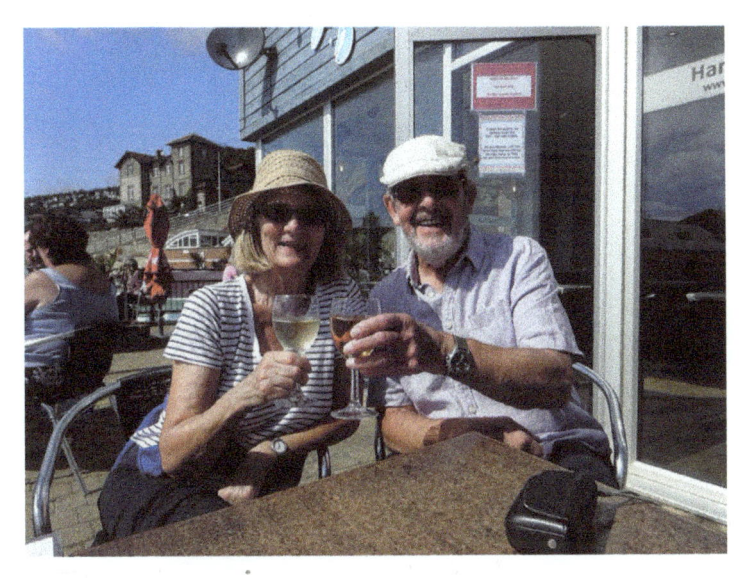

'Cheers! – RG and LB raise a glass to the Target Audience and the NHS – from their holiday destination of course.'

One fine day in the middle of a Covid night, RG and LB got up to fight; Back-to-back they faced each other, drew their swords and shot each other.

One was nearly blind and the other never sees, so, they sought a Target Audience mostly consisting of non-seeing and non-hearing referees!.

(anonymous but parts are gratefully borrowed).

Pete of dear friends Pat and Pete – who share RG and LB's love of Greece, on reading the first 'Dear Susan...' paperback remarked "a classic case of banging your head against a brick wall." This was after viewing an exhibition of John Craxton's Greek Odyssey on 14th October 2023 in Chichester. Pete and Craxton's paintings encouraged LB to bang his head a few more times for the sake of this sequel.

Over many years, RG and LB have had access to much of the Policy and Health Building documentation produced to guide the NHS. All this "Stupid Stuff" can be found in The British Library.

Without the pandemic and a spell in hospital for LB, they too would not have bothered to think about what might be done to help the NHS – but from now on they will always be on holiday.

A Short Letter to the RIBA Journal

Horrible Hospitals

Re 'Medical mutations' (RIBAJ, July, p38): I am not sure whether Christopher Shaw is speaking on behalf of Architects for Health or offering a personal view but my own opinion is that, following the first bout of Covid-19, we should avoid building 'European super hospitals' just as we should avoid if possible Covid-19. We should use those many hospital sites he mentions to build smarter, smaller hospitals that people (patients, their visitors and staff) can confidently access when they have to. These should be as unlike the nightmarish Nightingale hospitals as possible.

A large hospital is too big for patients and staff to comprehend and cannot be patient-focussed because its maze of rooms and corridors misinform, disorientate, and increase dependency. When it facilitates bad practice, it is not easily changed and because of its size and complexity, almost impossible to replace. Large hospitals have always become obsolete too soon and unmanageable for too long. We have had decades to understand this in project after project.

Len Bartholomew (former hospital planner and former member of Architects for Health)

August 2020

The Kings Fund press release of 13th February 2024 announcing its report calling for radical refocusing of the health and care system to put primary and community services at its core is worth a read as is its report. Unfortunately, this is more dire and as unreadable as LB's first 'Dear Susan...' paperback! (it did not warrant a mention in The Times on 14th February!). This report is unlikely to be implemented as it is also destined to be left on some faraway shore – or another crisis will come along to prevent its attempt at radical change. It is recommended reading as 'Another Last Word' even though it does not mention the obvious need to provide new, easy, fast, smart, smaller hospitals to replace failing large acute hospitals – when it should have done!

"We now need to plan our future hospital development on the basis of making essential provision for acute services in a way that will not pre-judge the eventual size of the district general hospitals. Fashions change: what is the conventional wisdom today may not be the wisdom tomorrow. By building for the essential, not the desirable number of beds, one can spread the limited capital resources and start more new hospital development."

Key note speech – Minister of Health, December 1975

Stop Press – March 2024

"Just 1 in 4 say NHS is working"

The Times front page – 27th March 2024

With reference to The British Social Attitudes Survey – September/October 2023, the Times Health Editor used this front-page article to indicate that "Approval rates have dropped to an historic low for almost all NHS services, including general practice, dentistry and hospitals."

The End

Dear Susan...

I'll say no more...
(thank you for listening)

LB

Milton Keynes UK
Ingram Content Group UK Ltd.
UKHW021034090524
442331UK00007B/96